Nursing Care Plans:

Nursing Diagnosis and Assessment, Nursing Interventions Guide

By

Brittany Samons

Table of Contents

Nursing Care Plans: Nursing Diagnosis and Assessment, Nursing Interventions Guide

By Brittany Samons

Introduction

As a nurse, you always have to be at your best. Diagnosing different medical conditions on sight and having plausible solutions to each problem could be the only thing between you and a life. Even though your training will rigorously take you through the remedies for the most common diseases, a frequent reminder on the latest symptoms and treatment options will not only keep you up to date but also ensure that you present the very best treatment services to your patients.

Experience is the best teacher. You will be well acquainted with the most common conditions in your area. However, there are the little random instances of a disease that will leave you clueless. While you always have the chance to consult, patients will always have more trust and better morale in someone who can act appropriately on impulse. Here are simple tips that will help you be that person to all your patients

1. Arthritis

Arthritis is a condition that develops with time. Arthritis makes simple routine tasks almost impossible to do as it affects the joints causing them to swell up and become painful. Fortunately, you can manage arthritis with the right treatment procedures.

Diagnosis and assessment

Proper diagnosis is the start of success treatment. Several symptoms must be considered in a physical exam such as movement of joints and extend of swollen joints. Sometimes blood tests and X-rays are needed to distinguish the exact type of arthritis a patient is suffering from. Sample fluid tests on infected joints will confirm the presence of arthritis as well as determine the right treatment approach.

Treatment/intervention

Treatment of arthritis aims at relieving pain and stiffness, as there is no treatment known to eliminate the condition. Medications in the form of ingestion drugs and cream applications are meant to slow down the disease progression. Occupational therapy is a great remedy for patients with arthritis.

2. Chronic Pain

Chronic pain treatment is a challenge. With the right combination however, it is possible to contain the condition. Choose a treatment that lasts between 2- 3 months or more. Early treatment also helps prevent pain from worsening.

Diagnosis and assessment

Pain is a personal experience and no tests can measure for sure how precise one's pain is. The best assessment is done based on the patient's description of the pain occurrence, its timing and location. Pain occurs in different parts of the body for different reasons hence the varied remedies.

Treatment/intervention

Chronic pain can be controlled in different ways as long as it improves the sufferer's condition. Common treatment options include acupuncture, meditation, nerve blocks, electric stimulation, and surgery. Relaxation therapies also help when dealing with pain. Some patients respond well to behavior modification treatment as a means of dealing with chronic pain.

Self-management of chronic pain is a promising treatment option too.

3. Liver Cirrhosis

The liver is the largest solid organ in the human body performing several important functions. When affected by cirrhosis the healthy tissue is replaced with scarred tissue, which hinder proper functioning of the liver. Blood flow is blocked thus hindering the processing of hormones, drugs and naturally produced toxins. Liver cirrhosis is ranked as one of the major death causing conditions in the world.

Diagnosis and Assessment

Obesity, chronic viral infections, blockage of the bile duct, repeated heart failure and specific diseases such as fibroid cysts and antitrypsin enzyme deficiency cause liver cirrhosis. Usually patients experience itchy skin, fatigue, fever, blood in stool, personality changes and sudden weight loss or gain. Blood tests, biopsy and physical exams can depict presence of the condition.

Intervention and treatment

Antiviral drugs and steroids may be used for treatment. Stopping alcohol abuse can also be a solution. In extreme cases, liver transplant may be required.

4. Tuberculosis

This potential fatal disease affects patients lungs. The causal bacteria is transferred through particles in coughs and sneezes. Its increased prevalence in developed countries is due to the spread of HIV, which weakens the immune system and ability to fight infection. Furthermore, different resistant strains have formed with time.

Diagnosis and assessment

TB has different symptoms including continuous coughing for more than three weeks. Patients cough blood, experience chest pains, fatigue, fever, night sweats, severe weight loss and loss of appetite as well as chills. Furthermore, this condition also affects other body parts including the brain, kidney and spine. You need to visit a medic in case you get in contact with an infected person, suffer from HIV, work around high risk persons and when using IV drugs.

Treatment/ intervention

Combination antibiotics are effective for the treatment of extra-pulmonary TB when administered for a period of 12 months. Latent TB where infection exists without symptoms should also be treated using a combination of rifampicin and isoniazid for three months.

5. Aspiration

Aspiration occurs when food liquid, vomit or saliva are breathed into the lungs or airways causing infection in the process. The bacterial infection depends on one's health, residence, status of hospitalization and antibiotic use in the past few days. There are different factors that could trigger the condition such as being less attentive due to medication, excessive drinking of alcohol, old age, anaesthesia among others.

Diagnosis and Assessment

There are certain symptoms you should be on the lookout for when suspecting aspiration. Bluish skin discoloration indicates lack of oxygen due to aspiration. Coughing smelly, green sputum or pus with blood, chest pain, fever, wheezing, excessive sweating and wheezing sounds are a few of the indicators. Some patients may have trouble swallowing.

Treatment/ intervention

Depending on the severity of the condition, patients may require hospitalization. A breathing machine may be used to support breathing. Antibiotics may also be administered.

6. Bleeding Risk

Internal bleeding occurs in different parts of the body causing excruciating pain in patients and sufferers. When suspected anticoagulation or antiplatelet medication are in order especially when properly balanced.

Diagnosis and assessment

Severe cases of internal bleeding leads to shock. This bleeding occurs within tissues, organs or in body cavities. The danger with internal bleeding is that it is difficult to diagnose since symptoms only show after a significant blood loss occurs translating to massive damage. Sometimes a blood clot large enough to compress an organ and interfere with its proper functioning can set off the alarm. Generally, the condition occurs when damaged arteries or veins allow blood to escape the circulatory system and accumulate in other body parts.

Intervention/ treatment

Blood-thinning medication is the most suitable for this condition. Anticoagulant medication such as heparin

and antiplatelet medication including aspirin and
clopidogrel can help treat bleeding risk.

7. Diarrhoea

Diarrhoea in most cases goes away after three days without treatment. However, in case it persist you may have to seek medical assistance. This is especially if lifestyle changes and home remedies seem not work.

Diagnosis and assessment

Diarrhoea is caused mainly by infection after being in contact with a person who has it. Food poisoning from taking contaminated food or drinks is another reason. Acute diarrhoea lasts a few days and clears on it on but the resistant chronic diarrhoea should be a cause for concern. Sometimes underlying conditions and medication types trigger diarrhoea.

Intervention and treatment

Different measures can be taken to contain the condition based on its extent of damage. The first treatment should be to remain hydrated through drinks and foods, treating underlying conditions and toning down on the drugs or changing them completely. Antibiotics usually work for diarrhoea but in some extreme cases where intestines may be removed, surgery is necessary.

8. Anxiety

Getting anxious is normal especially when faced with a challenging situation such as an interview or exam. It only becomes problematic when you have to worry about life problems constantly. The disorder manifest in different ways hence the varied types. Effective treatment is possible once you understand that anxiety is the body's natural response to danger, pressure and other stressful situations.

Diagnosis and assessment

A patient could have panic disorder, social anxiety disorder, general anxiety disorder, obsessive-compulsive disorder, posttraumatic disorder and phobia. All these forms of anxiety manifest in different forms. General symptoms are either physical or emotional. The common symptoms of the disorder are fatigue, insomnia, headaches, irritability, low concentration, and restlessness among other.

Intervention and treatment

An attack is bound to happen when a patient has muscle tension, hot flashes and chills or trembling.

Anxiety can be treated professionally through behavioural therapies including both cognitive and exposure therapies.

9. Asthma

This chronic disease affects the airways in the lungs. It results when the bronchus that allow air to pass in and out of the lungs are inflamed. The swelling causes muscles around to be tighten and as such, several symptoms are triggered.

Diagnosis and assessment

Look out for certain symptoms before qualifying the condition as asthma. Experts think that shortness of breath, chest tightening and pain, chronic coughing and trouble sleeping due to wheezing are some of the main symptoms. Sometimes asthma flare-ups are caused by allergens. To know for sure different tests must be conducted. Spirometry is one of the common breathing tests that asthma patients take as it indicates the functioning of the lungs. Allergy testing also comes into play with asthma patients.

Treatment/ intervention

Once asthma has been proven to exist, management is in order since no cure exists. It is important to take medication as advised. Combination inhalers, oral drugs and quick relief drugs are some of the medications a patient can be given.

10. Hypertension

Blood pressure measurements are given in two numbers, the systolic BP and diastolic BP.it is possible that either of the two numbers can be too high hence hypertension. It is important to keep checking your blood pressure readings to prevent any serious problems.

Diagnosis and assessment

Blood pressure can be measured when you visit the doctor or a medical clinic. Depending on the readings, it is possible to determine if your blood pressure is normal or hypertensive. In case of the second option, you will be able to know what stage you are. A medical practitioner needs to pay attention to both readings.

Treatment/ intervention

Lifestyle changes is a start when you want to contain your hypertension. However, there is need for additional treatment to lower the pressure to a normal state. The drug/ medication administered depends on the patient's age. Beta-blockers, thiazide diuretics, renin inhibitors as well as calcium channel blockers are some of the prescriptions a hypertensive patient can get.

11. Breast Cancer

Ore breast cancer patients today are getting improved care due to increased awareness of the condition. Unlike some time back, information is available and the scourge around breast cancer is slowly diminishing. Patients are increasingly getting sport, which is important for their recovery.

Diagnosis and assessment

Breast cancer is diagnosed in different forms:

Self-evaluation where patient notices an abnormal lump in the breast

Mammogram: This is a low dose x-ray of the breast, which allows the radiologist to notice any abnormalities accurately

Breast ultrasound: This helps to determine if the lump on the breast is a fluid filled cyst or solid cyst

Breast MRI: This is only recommended for specific breast cancer situations because of the injection used

Breast biopsy: Involves sampling the affected region before making a conclusive diagnosis

Intervention/ treatment

Treatments include chemotherapy, radiotherapy and use of mediation to contain treatment related side effects.

12. Bulimia Nervosa

Every person has had struggles with food turning to it when stressed. Bulimia nervosa on the other hand is more like a compulsion to eat excess food and exercising to get rid of it. Your body takes a toll on the eating and purging routine and without treatment it can be fatal.

Diagnosis and assessment

Patients suffering from bulimia always show specific signs that doctors and medical practitioners can use to diagnose the problem. These include:

Lack of control to overeating

Secrecy around the eating environment

Consuming unusually large amounts of foods

Alternating between fasting and overeating

Calluses and scars on fingers

Frequent weight fluctuations

Interventions/ treatment

Patients should be advised to seek psychological help to boost their self-worth and low esteems. They also should stay away from areas that bring temptation to indulge in food. Bulimia therapy is one of the most effective treatments available.

13. Leukemia

Early diagnosis and treatment of leukemia is almost impossible because there are no constant signs for all forms of the disease. You need to visit a doctor immediately in case you notice swollen gums and lymph nodes for proper diagnosis.

Diagnosis and assessment

Physical examinations involving checking for enlarged lymph nodes and enlarged liver and spleen among other things is one of the test that a doctor can conduct. There is also blood testing that will show abnormal white cell count and assist in the diagnosis of leukemia. Needle biopsy and pelvic bone marrow aspiration will have to be carried out for the specific leukemia type to be sure what type of leukemia a patient is suffering from.

Intervention/ treatment

Advancements in medical technology makes it possible for leukemia patients to survive longer. Possible treatments include chemotherapy, blood and platelets transfusion to prevent blood loss and medications to control related side effects.

14. Diabetes

Certain risk factors are what will make your doctor suspect that you have diabetes. High levels of sugars in your urine is one of the first triggers. This could be so because you have little or no insulin as the pancreas fails to produce.

Diagnosis and assessment

Proper diagnosis of diabetes is crucial for containing the condition before it gets out of hand. Three tests can be conducted namely:

Fasting glucose test that tests blood sugar levels and is taken first thing in the morning before you eat

Oral glucose tolerance test where patients drink beverage containing glucose the blood sugar levels taken within the first half hour to one hour.

A1c tests that shows the average blood sugar levels for the past 2-3 months

Intervention/ treatment

You need a treatment plan from your doctor. You may have to work with a team of healthcare professionals.

There is need to closely monitor blood sugar levels especially when taking insulin doses.

15. Migraines

Severe headaches that come with feelings of nausea, vomiting and sensitivity to light among other symptoms is common. Some patients have warning signs before the actual migraines come. It is only with proper diagnosis that suitable treatment can follow.

Diagnosis and assessment

Visiting a qualified doctor when you experience constant headaches is important. You need to be sure that the headaches are not a sign of an underlying serious problem. Medical experts will use your medical history to make a conclusive diagnosis. Sometimes CAT and MRI scans may be done to know exactly what part of your brain triggers the migraines. Make sure you have a detailed outline of your treatment.

Intervention/ treatment

Patients should avoid potential triggers such as foods and stress. This is the reason why keeping a record of attacks is important. Patients are either given abortive or prophylactic treatments to control and prevent symptoms respectively.

16. Lower Back Pain

Younger people between the age of thirty and sixty years are likely to suffer more from lower back pain due to the strain or the disc spaces. The causes are suspected to be from a possible muscle strain or ligament strain after lifting heavy objects, sudden twisting and development of microscopic tears.

Diagnosis and assessment

Lower back pain can be complex to diagnose because of the many structures in the spine that are likely to cause pain. Most doctors ask patients to describe the location of the pain, severity as well as the type of pain they are experiencing for them to assess. Acknowledging that even though no known anatomical cause of back pain exists this does not eliminate the existence of pain.

Intervention/ treatment

Patients are advised to take a lot of rest for the injured tissues to heal. Medications from over the counter to prescriptions drugs are also available.

17. Parkinson's Disease

This chronic movement disorder with no known cause and cure. Most people live with the disease. The malfunctioning and death of neurons in the brain triggers production of dopamine, which sends a message to other parts of the brain controlling movements.

Diagnosis and assessments

The symptoms of PD vary from one patient to the next. Doctors and specialist base their assessments and diagnosis on the following symptoms:

Tremors of the hands, arms, legs, jaw and faces
Rigidity of the limbs and trunk
Postural instability
Slow movement

Seeking the assistance of qualified medical practitioners is the only way to diagnose the problem early.

Intervention/ treatment

There are many treatment options available for this conditional though none can reverse the symptoms. The best a patient can do is manage the symptoms by taking different drugs during the day. The options of treatment include:

Over the counter medication

Prescription drugs

Surgical treatments

18. Pneumonia

Inflammation of the air sacs in both lungs is the cause of pneumonia especially if it fills up with fluid or pus. A number of things including fungi, bacteria and pneumonia causes this condition. Pneumonia ranges from mild to life threatening hence early diagnosis and treatment is necessary.

Diagnosis and Assessment

Common symptoms of pneumonia include sharp chest pain, excessive sweating, loss of appetite and fever. This condition can be diagnosed through a number of ways including:

Physical examinations, a medic listens to the lungs with a stethoscope

Chest x-rays

A range of tests including sputum, CBC blood tests and pleural fluid culture

Pulse oximetry, bronchoscopy, and CT scans can also be done.

Treatment/ intervention

Treatment depends on the type of pneumonia. Nurses can administer cough treatment but should refer patients in case breathing treatment is involved. Antibiotics may also be administered under the prescription of a doctor.

19. Alzheimer's Disease

Alzheimer is a disease that affects the brain. This condition worries people over the age of 55 years and can be a great cause for emotional stress. Most people assume that because they forget things they could be suffering from Alzheimer's which is not the case and only proper diagnosis can identify the disease.

Diagnosis and assessment

Certain symptoms can easily help you diagnose the condition. Some of these signs include:

Routinely forgetting where you placed important items because you put them in odd places

Frequently forgetting entire conversations

Forgetting or inappropriately replacing names of common objects and family members

Rapid mood change and cancellation dates with friends and family

Intervention and treatment

Mist forms of treatments are based on clinical trials. However the diseases can be managed in different ways most of which target containing the symptoms especially mood swings.

20. Heart Attack

The heart muscle requires constant supply of oxygen for nourishment. The coronary artery supplies the necessary oxygen to the heart. In case of coronary artery diseases, less bloods goes to the heart and triggers heart attack.

Diagnosis and assessment

Before a heart attack happens patients are likely to feel undue fatigue, experience difficulties in breathing, chest discomforts, as well as palpitations. It is important that the disease be diagnosed in good time. For this, the doctor will have to do a few things.

Conduct a physical examination

Go through the patient's medical history

Carry out an electrocardiogram test that discovers abnormalities and damages to the heart.

Blood testing to detect abnormal enzyme levels in the blood

Intervention / treatment

Thrombolysis – injection of a clot dissolving agent to restore blood flow in the coronary artery

Coronary artery bypass graft surgery- suitable in case thrombolysis is not done immediately

21. Pancreatitis

The condition where the pancreas gets inflamed is serious considering its importance in digestion. The damage occurs when the enzymes are activated before they are released into the small intestines and begin attacking the pancreas.

Diagnosis and assessment

Doctors diagnose this condition by measuring the level of two enzymes in the blood. High levels of amylase and lipase indicate the presence of acute pancreatitis. Apart from blood tests, doctors conduct other tests to diagnose. These include:

Pancreatic function check to discover if the pancreas is generating the proper amount of digestive enzymes

Glucose tolerant test that measures damaged cells if the pancreas that make insulin

CT scan and ultra sound

ERCP that looks at the bile duct using X-rays

Intervention/ treatment

The most common treatment for acute pancreatitis is using IV fluids and pain relievers when the patient is hospitalized. Surgery is needed for severe cases.

22. Autism

A neurodevelopment disorder affecting the sufferer's ability to communicate and socially relate with others. This disease is more prevalent in boys than girls are. No two people suffering from autism are the same making the condition unique to handle. Mild disorders cannot be recognized until later in life.

Diagnosis and assessment

Due to the difference in manifestation, autism cannot be diagnosed equally in all patients. Sometimes autism screen may be used where short yes or no answers will help determine if the disorder is present. Parent reports and direct observations are important when making diagnosis. Clinicians may inquire from peers and school in case the child in question is older.

Interventions /Treatments

No cure exists for autism. However, with educational therapies some of the symptoms may reduce. ABA is one of the most effective treatment therapies mediation can be used to reduce irritation but cannot be used to reduce core symptoms.

23. Flu

The only way to know if what you are experiencing is flu is to observe certain symptoms such as cough, sore throat, headaches, fatigue and runny or stuffy noses. This disease occurs mostly during the rainy and dry season due to the allergens and causal agents. However, doctors can tell for sure if you have flu by testing.

Diagnosis and assessment

Influenza virus can be detected in a number of ways. Rapid influenza diagnostic tests is the most commonly used test probably because it brings result after 30 minutes. Its efficiency is however questionable as it sometimes gives negatives when you have the flu. More sensitive and accurate results can be conducted in specialized laboratories. Clinical judgment and symptoms are also simple ways that this condition can be diagnosed.

Intervention / treatment

Patients should be advised to rest, drink fluids to avoid dehydration, take pain relievers and cough syrups as prescribed by the medic.

24. Ectopic Pregnancy

When a fertilized egg fails to move to the uterus for attachment and remains in the fallopian tube, ectopic pregnancy develops causing complications. These pregnancies put the lives of mothers at risk and require emergency treatment. It is mostly discovered at the eighth week of pregnancy.

Diagnosis and assessment

Ectopic pregnancies are sad because only in rare cases does the mother and child survive. t is important that it is diagnosed early to help minimize the pain of loss. Doctors can observe symptoms such as light vaginal bleeding, painful nausea and vomiting, lower abdominal pains, dizziness and weakness as well as shoulder and back pain. When the fallopian tube rupture the pain becomes severe and could lead to fainting.

Intervention/ treatment

Treatment includes observation, laparoscopy, and medication. Sometimes ectopic pregnancies will resolve on their own without intervention and the patient needs to advise to wait out especially if the condition is not severe.

Final Words

Nursing patients back to health depends on your ability to identify conditions and sort them out as soon as possible. Being ready for each problem your daily professional life might throw at you will make you a better nurse. Sometimes, the doctor might not be near to help you sort out the problems. At such times, it is up to you to dig deep into your knowledge and come up with the best solutions to the problem at hand.

Understanding that medical conditions keep on changing, and so do their treatments is a motivator enough to keeping on learning new tricks. Staffing your locker with the most commonly used medication should increase your response time since having the information without the tools you need to implement it is equally useless. Go through the document every now and then to refresh your memory. Better still, you can do it in a group with your colleagues to ensure that the entire team is always at its best at all times.

Thank You Page

I want to personally thank you for reading my book. I hope you found information in this book useful and I would be very grateful if you could leave your honest review about this book. I certainly want to thank you in advance for doing this.

If you have the time, you can check my other books too.

Printed in the USA
CPSIA information can be obtained
at www.ICGtesting.com
CBHW060001020224
3960CB00015B/1043